YOUR KNOWLEDGE HAS VALUE

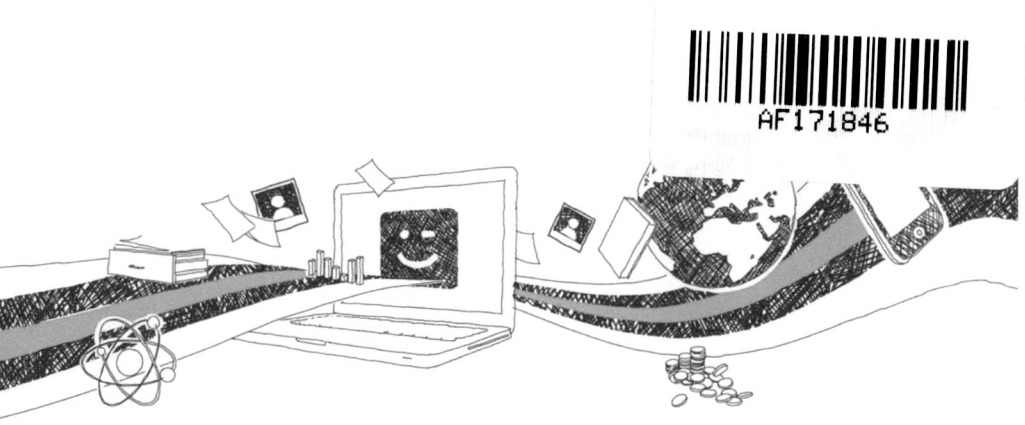

- We will publish your bachelor's and master's thesis, essays and papers

- Your own eBook and book - sold worldwide in all relevant shops

- Earn money with each sale

Upload your text at www.GRIN.com and publish for free

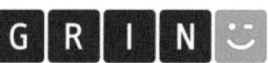

Bibliographic information published by the German National Library:

The German National Library lists this publication in the National Bibliography; detailed bibliographic data are available on the Internet at http://dnb.dnb.de .

This book is copyright material and must not be copied, reproduced, transferred, distributed, leased, licensed or publicly performed or used in any way except as specifically permitted in writing by the publishers, as allowed under the terms and conditions under which it was purchased or as strictly permitted by applicable copyright law. Any unauthorized distribution or use of this text may be a direct infringement of the author s and publisher s rights and those responsible may be liable in law accordingly.

Imprint:

Copyright © 2017 GRIN Verlag
Print and binding: Books on Demand GmbH, Norderstedt Germany
ISBN: 9783668629936

This book at GRIN:

https://www.grin.com/document/384453

Patrick Kimuyu

Impact of Hybrid Technology in the Operating Room

GRIN Verlag

GRIN - Your knowledge has value

Since its foundation in 1998, GRIN has specialized in publishing academic texts by students, college teachers and other academics as e-book and printed book. The website www.grin.com is an ideal platform for presenting term papers, final papers, scientific essays, dissertations and specialist books.

Visit us on the internet:

http://www.grin.com/

http://www.facebook.com/grincom

http://www.twitter.com/grin_com

Impact of Hybrid Technology in the Operating Room

Patrick Kimuyu

Contents

Introduction 2
Literature Review 3
    IMRI 3
    Endovascular 4
    Computed Tomography (CT) 5
    Angiography 5
Recommendations and Future Directions 6
Conclusion 8
References List 9

Introduction

Over the decades, technological advancement in medical technology has advanced to ensure that experts in the operating rooms such as radiographers, anesthesiologists, and surgeons work collaboratively to produce effective results. The components of a hybrid suite call for a suite that is large enough to accommodate the required equipment in reference to the kind of intervention technique. The hybrid technology is a novice avenue to new diagnostic and treatment possibilities and has taken minimally invasive medical procedures to a new level. Huynh and Bechara (2013) note that hybrid interventions are integral to limb revascularization procedures, accounting for 5% to 21% of all these procedures. The hybrid equipment is flexible in that they can be integrated into the case of operative procedures as well as stand-alone components as shown in the CT section. Therefore, this literature review focuses on creating understanding on the impact of hybrid technology in the operating room.

Significance of Hybrid Technology

The hybrid technology in the operating room merges two distinct and different areas to yield effective results. The essence of this new technology in medicine is to substitute invasive procedures with minimally invasive ones based on empirical evidence on their efficacy and long-term benefits. Hudorović et al. (2010) note that these hybrid procedures are associated with reduced morbidity and mortality rates, and especially among the elderly as they are largely exposed to operative morbidity and mortality. In the recent years, the increase in the use of hybrid procedures has increased, and especially in reference to CT scans (Huynh & Bechara, 2013). There is no standard hybrid procedure but the more dynamic the operating room, the better its efficacy; but, there is a need for standard clinical guidelines for this hybrid technology.

There are various hybrid treatment procedures in light of the condition being treated. However, this paper concentrates on the hybrid technologies that integrate the imaging component to ensure that definitive treatment is administered (Kataoka et al., 2016). In reference to available literature, the most common hybrid imaging techniques are those that employ computer tomography (CT) and angiography to view vascular anatomy, orthopedic trauma, and various kinds of tumors in view that cardiovascular, injuries, and cancers are among the most common conditions.

Literature Review

The hybrid treatment method composed of a combination of emergency surgery and interventional radiology(IVR) is perceived to be an ideal strategy for treating severely injured patients in the operating room because it reduces the time of resuscitation and treatment (Kataoka et al., 2016). Considering that the efficacy of this mode of treatment has not been adequately researched, Kataoka et al., (2016) set out to determine the efficacy of IVR that includes a mobile digital subtraction angiography (DSA) combined the emergency surgery when administered to individuals with severe trauma. The research by Kataoka et al., (2016) indicated that hybrid treatment is an effective type of treatment in increasing overall survival. In addition, this mode of treatment was found to be effective in reducing therapeutic damage and preserving organ functions as well as tissue planes. IVR aided in damage control because it controlled hemorrhage when definitive repair proved ineffective.

The application of transarterial embolization (TAE) in the control of arterial hemorrhage in tandem with damage control surgery was found to be effective inhemodynamically unstable patients who have gone through trauma. The surgical procedures used in this study included craniotomy, laparotomy, hemostasis, damage control surgery, and thoracotomy. However, this study was a retrospective one based on hospital records; hence, it is bound to have been affected by bias considering that the procedures had been conducted by different healthcare workers and some subjective elements to the provision of care cannot be accounted. This study is a good basis for future studies because it lacks the methodological rigor required when control and intervention groups are used. Thereby the essence of this particular study whose essence will be to use a randomized controlled trial to determine the causal effect of hybrid treatment as opposed to theadministration of IVR and surgery is isolation; even though they are both administered, their application does not render them as hybrid kind of treatment.

Interventional techniques used in hybrid operation suites for the purposes of enhancing imaging are discussed below (Hudorović et al., 2010; Rogostki et al., 2012; Crowhurst, Campbell, Whitby & Pathmanathan, 2013; Tanaka et al., 2014; Tan et al., 2015).

IMRI

Intraoperative Magnetic Resonance Imaging combines operative procedures with MRI to produce efficient intraoperative evaluation methods to review cerebral interventions and resections. Obtaining a precise and accurate MRI during an operative procedure is imperative because it directs the healthcare team to further resections and more interventions without wasting time and using additional resources associated with the transfer of a patient to a suitable location. When a hybrid environment in reference to IMR lacks, there is adelay,and the entire procedure tends to take longer than expected. This realization is only theorized, and there are insufficient studies to prove these hypotheses (Rogoski et al., 2012). Apparently, the sterile operating room is not a suitable environment for magnetic fields, which require high safety precautions; hence, the need for relocating the patient and this interferes with the efficiency of the entire procedure. However, by allowing surgical interventions and MRI examinations to take place simultaneously, evaluation and required interventions use minimal time. Considering that there are two approaches through IMRI suites can be set-up, there are no guidelines to indicate for which procedures are ideal for the two types of scanners: fixed and mobile. Research is required to relate the types of medical procedures or conditions to the most favorable scanner (Rogoski et al., 2012).

Endovascular

Endovascular technology has progressively evolved into a less invasive method that is used to treat vascular disease. This technology began in 1996 when a mini-invasive approach that entailed the combination of "left anterior small thoracotomy and percutaneous transluminal coronary angioplasty" was used as a staging treatment technique or postoperative intervention for individuals with heart disease (Tan et al., 2015). Also, this technology has been used a hybrid technique entailing the combination of endovascular technique and open surgery as a treatment mode for subclavian artery injuries.

Endovascular techniques are indicated to be an effective alternative to open surgical repair in the treatment of vascular injury. Hudorović et al., (2010) note that the vascular hybrid room requires various equipment to ensure it yields the intended outcomes. Therefore, a C-arm, special imaging table, booms, surgical lights, advanced communication systems to relay information on surgical and radiological images when and where needed as well as flat panel arms and displays. An endovascular operating suite composed of all these components enables conversion when necessary to allow the change from a sterile environment to a magnetic one without exposing the patient to infections as he or she is transported from one room to another. During endovascular interventions, an on-table duplex ultrasound is useful for making puncturing easy as well as guiding the endovenous laser therapy (Hudorović et al., 2010). The imaging component in a vascular hybrid room is useful in producing images of superior quality, measurement abilities for procedures of high resolution, and provides tube heat capacities of higher degrees (Hudorović et al., 2010).

Endovascular treatments have been found to be effective in reference to injuries of the aorta, major veins, and peripheral arteries. Instead of an open surgical method, stent or stent-graft placement has been found to be more effective in the repair of conduit vessel lesions. The use of hybrid endovascular treatment for the various vascular procedures has been shown to require reduced radiation dosage without affecting the course of treatment; hence proving to be more effective and reliable (Hertault et al., 2014; van den Haak, Hamans, Zuurmond, Verhoeven, & Koning, 2015). The treatment of abdominal aortic aneurysms (AAA) has shifted from the use of surgical procedures to endovascular ones. Literature suggests that some endovascular intervention entails an angiography component (Tanaka et al., 2014). A historical approach to endovascular techniques indicates that hybrid interventions in the operating room use mobile fluoroscopy together with digital subtraction angiography.

Computed Tomography (CT)

CT goes be various names in various literal works, including angiographic CT, C-arm CT, volume CT, and rotational angiography. The use of computed tomography is essential to a hybrid suite because it helps to add on to the capabilities of the operation suite by enhancing access to high-quality digital subtraction (Crowhurst et al., 2013). Also, three-dimensional imaging is available when needed. Examples of hybrid CT scanners include the Single Photon Emission Computed Tomography (SPECT/CT) and Positron Emission Tomography (PET/CT). Both of these interventional procedures can be used as part of the hybrid technology as well as independent entities for use during conventional procedures (Johnson, 2016). The combination of CT and angiography is useful in the management of occlusive arterial disease I view that the decision for reconstruction is governed by clinical judgment. Huynh and Bechara (2013) indicate that close to 25% of patients require a combination of both aortoiliac and infrainguinalrevascularization; hence, it is important to accurately identify these patients using the hybrid CT/angiography system.

Angiography

When 3D angiography properties are fitted in an operating room, it becomes easier to perform operational procedures because an individual's vascular anatomy is more visible. This kind of technology in operating procedures is ideal for "coronary, peripheral, or cerebral vascular procedures." Even though this is an under-researched area, the effects of the hybrid technology cannot be ignored. An angiography unit can be used simultaneously with other interventional techniques, such as endovascular procedures and CT. Thereby; it becomes possible to apply all the required treatment techniques without moving a patient and compromising the sterile conditions. In addition, such a hybrid intervention prevents needle and catheter dislocation. The combination of an angiography unit and CT has been used for various oncologic procedures. Also, a study by Tsagakis et al. (2013) indicate the combined use of angiography and CT on cardiological patients as well to yield positive results associated with reduced mortality due to accurate diagnosis and design of prompt treatment. In the article by Crowhurst et al., (2013), the authors discuss the use of the hybrid CT and angiography system in the detection of hepatocellular carcinoma. This detection technique includes the application of two techniques: CT arterio-portography (CTAP) and CT hepatic arteriography (CTHA).

Most of the empirical research is based on case studies, whose results are not generalizable or from hospital records that were not obtained using clearly laid down research methods. The role of the angiographic unit, in reference to the reviewed literature, is versatile as it is used in combination with many interventional procedures. When used simultaneously with open surgery, it enhanced the performance of IVR procedures. Minimally invasive vascular procedures are currently being adapted to treat peripheral artery disease (PAD) using percutaneous interventions and emerging angiogenesis as well as advanced molecular genetics to replace arterial revascularization (Hudorović et al., 2010).

This technology can also be used alongside CT to achieve superselective transarterial chemoembolization (TACE) of hepatocellular carcinoma (HCC) to determine tumor-feeding arteries and make predictions about embolization areas. This hybrid method is associated with prolonged survival for patients with this carcinoma because this hybrid method helps to ax processes that promote tumor growth. The combined use of angiography and CT is indicated to be better than the use of CT alone in a hybrid operating suite because the CT/angiography system has a high-contrast resolution of CT, large field of view, minimal artifacts, and is applies real-time CT fluoroscopy (Tanaka et al., 2015).

Recommendations and Future Directions

The hybrid technology is shown to be an effective method for providing quality care, but the implementation of this technology in hospitals requires a mixture of variant skills and knowledge if expected clinical outcomes are to be achieved (Kopelman, Lanzafame, & Kopelman, 2013). The literature review discussed above gives insight into the essence of the hybrid technology in the medical world, and in light to the radiology field, in the pursuit of efficiency in performance and effectiveness of the involved procedures. The hybrid technology is still a kind of new technology that has not yet been scaled up in all healthcare institutions, but the literature has confirmed that the method is beneficial though more conclusive empirical studies are required. The literature search revealed that hybrid technology is effective in an array of ways including attenuating delay of procedures and reducing the number of anesthesia given as patients are transferred from one location to the next to undergo different procedures at different places. Thereby, incorporating the relatively technology in the hospital would help in the delivery of effective services characterized by accuracy, convenience, and teamwork.

Despite the fact that it is a new technology that proves to be effective in delivery of quality healthcare services, its integration into the healthcare processes of the hospital can pose a huge challenge as employees resist change. First, employees are not knowledgeable about it, and it would require more than just documenting; radiologists would have to work collaboratively with the surgery team, and this requires a great deal of team spirit. For example, angiography and CT are ideal in the provision of vascular interventions and identifying orthopedic trauma (Crowhurst et al., 2013). The application the hybrid technology in the operating room requires collaboration among all the involved healthcare workers. Even though the guidelines for the implementation of this novice technology are yet to be developed, there is need to determine the level of intensity during imaging considering that being precise is paramount. Also, identifying the advantages and disadvantages of various hybrid technologies is important to determine their selection and when they should be applied, appropriately. These requirements for the new technology prove demanding to an individual, and the fear of trying out something new and the requirement for certain skills would result in the resistance to the novice hybrid technology. The hospital, therefore, needs to plan for a training program to educate its radiologists as plans to implement the new technology continue.

Prompt action to train its radiologists will save the hospital from using unnecessary resources planning for a recruitment process. Also, the hospital will not have to undergo shortage of staff because training of staff will go on as implementation plans are underway. Hence, by the time the installation process of the machines and a convenient suite are complete, a section of the staff members will be adequately knowledgeable to aid the others, who will undergo training at certain intervals times and the radiologists can learn from each other. Before all the radiologists can gain the confidence of working alone, they can work in twos. After deliberations and successfully learning the new system to accurately advise and work collaboratively with the healthcare team performing surgery, then radiologists can learn to work independently. Nonetheless, mobilization and pooling of resources to purchase the necessary machines and structure the operation suite in a recommendable style are important. Investing in this new technology is worth it because it is an opportunity for taking healthcare to another level intended to improve operative outcomes and associated quality of life because efficiency is associated with reduced hospital stays.

Conclusion

A hybrid operational suite is an effective and advanced area that helps to improve the performance of healthcare workers because diagnosis and treatment can be done concurrently without any delay in either of the procedures. As a radiographer, there is need to advance my skills because hybrid imaging is no longer a standalone modality but one that requires me to function across the various interventional modalities. Thereby, they need to work hand in hand with the operating healthcare team to ensure that my role is well played out so that images are produced timely as the surgical procedures proceed. Even though the use of imaging equipment is deemed effective in a hybrid suite, a radiographer needs to be aware of the dosage required considering the fact that operational procedures are in progress. A study by van den Haak et al. (2015) indicate a potential for reduced doses when hybrid technology is used, and there is need for radiographers to get these dosages right when this new technology is underway. Hence, there is limited x-ray exposure because imaging is accurate and well directed in view of collaborative teamwork. Thereby, having good background knowledge of the hybrid technology is necessary because, as a radiographer, Radiographer can advise doctors on how to go about an operative procedure without delaying operative interventions.

References List

Crowhurst, J. A., Campbell, D., Whitby, M., and Pathmanathan, P., 2013. Novel utilization of 3D technology and the hybrid operating theatre: Perioperative assessment of posterior sternoclavicular dislocation using cone beam CT. *Journal of Medical Radiation Sciences.* **60**(2), pp. 67-70.

Hertault, A., et al., 2014. Impact of hybrid rooms with image fusion on radiation exposure during endovascular aortic repair. *European Journal of Vascular and Endovascular Surgery.* **48**(4), pp. 382-390.

Hudorović, N., et al., 2010. The vascular hybrid room-operating room of the future. *Acta Clin Croat.* **49**(3), pp. 289-298.

Huynh, T.T. and Bechara, C.F., 2013. Hybrid interventions in limb salvage. *Methodist DeBakey Cardiovascular Journal.* **9**(2), pp. 90-94.

Kataoka, Y., et al., 2016. Hybrid treatment combining emergency surgery and intraoperative interventional radiology for severe trauma. *Injury.* **47**(1), pp. 59-63.

Kopelman, Y., Lanzafame, R.J. and Kopelman, D., 2013. Trends in evolving technologies in the operating room of the future. *JSLS : Journal of the Society of Laparoendoscopic Surgeons.* **17**(2), pp. 171-173.

Tan, H., et al., 2015. "One-Stop Hybrid Procedure" in the Treatment of Vascular Injury of Lower Extremity. *Indian Journal of Surgery.* **77**(1), pp. 75-78.

Tsagakis, K., et al., 2013. Hybrid operating room concept for combined diagnostics, intervention and surgery in acute type: A dissection. *European Journal of Cardio-Thoracic Surgery : Official Journal of the European Association for Cardio-Thoracic Surgery.* **43**(2), pp. 397-404.

Van den haak, R., et al., 2015. Significant radiation dose reduction in the hybrid operating room using a novel X-ray imaging technology. *European Journal of Vascular and Endovascular Surgery.* **50**(4), pp. 480-486.

YOUR KNOWLEDGE HAS VALUE

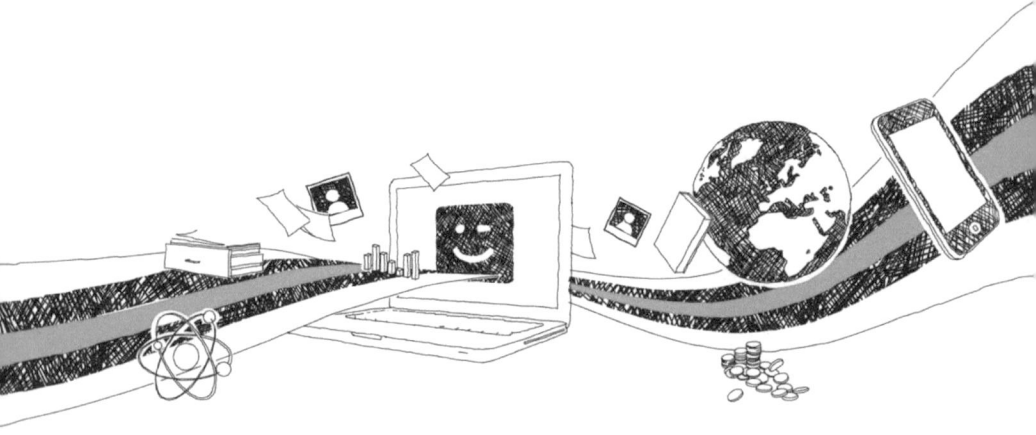

- We will publish your bachelor's and master's thesis, essays and papers

- Your own eBook and book - sold worldwide in all relevant shops

- Earn money with each sale

Upload your text at www.GRIN.com and publish for free

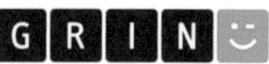